50 DELICIOUS SLOW COOKER RECIPES

Just Assemble Your Dish, Relax and Allow All the Gorgeous Flavors to Meld Over Low Heat.

Slow Cooking Academy

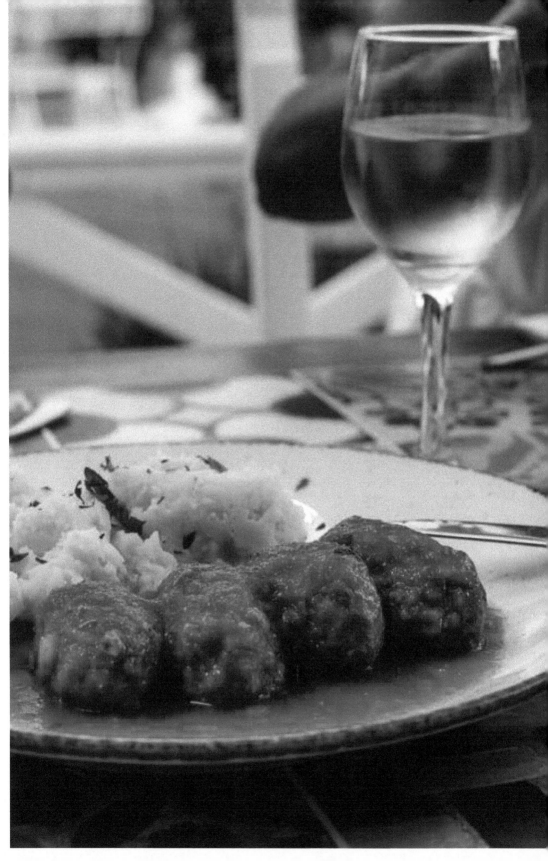

liable for any hardship or damages that may befall them after undertaking the information described herein.

Additionally, the information in the following pages is intended only for informational purposes and should thus be thought of as universal. As befitting its nature, it is presented without assurance regarding its prolonged validity or interim quality. Trademarks that are mentioned are done without written consent and can in no way be considered an endorsement from the trademark holder.

Table of Contents

INTRODUCTION

The slow cooker, or crockpot, is an appliance that simmers food at a low temperature. A variety of dishes can be prepared in a crockpot, but the results will be different from baking, boiling, or frying. It was introduced to the world in 1950 and at that time was named Simmer Crock. This book will describe how crockpots are used, the various designs and how they operate. We will discuss the benefits and drawbacks to this handy appliance.

Why Slow Cooker Meals?

The crockpot was given its name in 1971 after modifications were made to the original design. A crockpot is oval or round in shape, contains buttons or dials for control, and has a digital timer. The cooking pot has a lid that is often made of glass. It is usually made of ceramic with a glaze that is used to seal the inherent porosity of earthenware with a surrounding metal container. The ceramic pot acts as a cooking dish and heat reservoir at the same time. A crockpot can hold from 500 ml to 7 liters, depending on its design. It usually had cooking settings (low, medium, or high) and a keep warm setting.

The food to be cooked is placed within the pot with some liquid which may or may not need to be pre-heated. Once it reaches its set temperature, it will remain constant while the food is cooked. If you are adapting a recipe for your slow cooker, you might want to add some liquid in case of evaporation.

Benefits of a crockpot

- A crockpot replaces the need for several pans. Everything is put in the pot and cooks together.
- A crockpot cooks food in a completely covered atmosphere so all the ingredients can fully blend. This enriches the flavors of the ingredients and gives a delicious taste to the food.
- It is convenient to use because you do not have to constantly monitor the dish. You can put your ingredients in the pot and come back after several hours to a delicious meal.
- Keep food inside the crockpot moist by adding sufficient liquid or sauce. This is good for cooking cheap cuts of meat like beef chuck, pork shoulder, or brisket.
- If you have several dishes to make, using a crockpot for one will cut down on the number of pans and allow you to make more than one thing at a time.
- A crockpot consists of a porcelain layer and a metal housing which nicely traps all heat inside. The heat stays inside the pot and does not burn or heat up its surroundings.

- Because a crockpot closes tightly, it not only retains heat, but it also prevents boiling dry and burning.
- Crockpots work at a low temperature, which means they use a minimum amount of energy, much less than an electric oven.
- Because of its low cooking temperature, food cooked in a crockpot does not scorch.
- Crockpot cooking is very easy, usually just one or two steps. All you need to do is place your ingredients in the pot, put on the lid, and press set.

Tips and Tricks for Slow Cooker Success

1. Add the Right Amount of Food

One of our most important slow cooker cooking tips: Put the appropriate amount of food in the slow cooker before turning it on, making sure the cooker is at least half full but no more than two-thirds full.

2. Layer It Correctly

Bottom to top: vegetables, meat, and then liquid. Cut potatoes, carrots, parsnips and other dense vegetables into small pieces before placing them in the slow cooker. These heavier, fresh greens make a great base at the bottom of your pot. Tender vegetables like zucchini, broccoli, green beans, or peas are best added toward the end of cooking.

3. Don't Use Frozen Uncooked Meat

Never start with frozen raw meat as bacteria grow quickly in the 40-140°F danger zone. Frozen meat does not reach a safe temperature quickly enough and stays in the danger zone too long to be safe to consume. Defrost meat in the refrigerator overnight or for as long as needed to avoid frozen spots.

4. Dairy and seafood go in last!

Dairy and seafood will break down if they sit in the slow cooker for too long, so always remember that seafood should be added in the last hour of cooking, and dairy within the last 15 minutes.

5. No peeking or stirring!

You might be curious about what's going on inside the crockpot, but opening that lid is a no-no. Every time you do, you're adding up to 20 minutes additional cooking time. If you really feel the need to glance inside and check for doneness, the ideal time is 30-45 minutes before the end of the cooking time.

Slow Cooker Food Safety

- **Do not cook dry beans**

Soak and pre-cook dried beans before adding to your recipe. Dried beans contain a natural toxin which is easily destroyed by boiling temperatures. Soak the beans for 12 hours, rinse, and then cook for at least 10 minutes before putting the beans in a slow cooker.

- **Do not cook frozen foods**

Make sure frozen meat or vegetables are properly thawed before putting them in the slow cooker. Adding these ingredients to the mixture while they are still frozen can pose a serious health risk, because leaving the food in a dangerous temperature zone is a magnet for bacteria.

- **Store leftovers in shallow containers and refrigerate within two hours**

Make sure you are storing them safely and eating them in a timely manner to reduce the risk of food poisoning. Store leftovers in shallow containers and refrigerate within two hours of removing from the pot.

Smart Plan Ahead Makes Slow Cooking Easier

Read the entire recipe and gather all the ingredients (and required equipment) before and start cooking. It will save you the frustration of finding out you doesn't have potatoes in your pantry.

- Put frozen foods in the refrigerator to defrost them the day before cooking.
- Menu-plan for the week to help you remember when to thaw frozen meat or something else.
- If you're constantly in a rush in the morning, prepare some or all parts of the recipe the night before. Store the food in an airtight container in the refrigerator, and then pop it into the slow cooker in the morning, set the timer, and off you go.

BREAKFAST

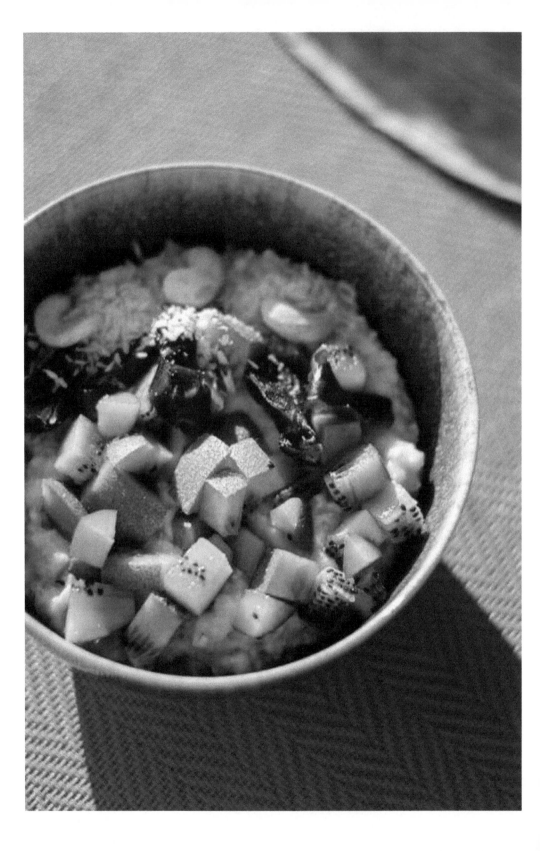

Tomato Hot Eggs

5 Servings

Preparation Time: 2.5 hours 10 minutes

Ingredients

- 1 teaspoon Coconut oil
- 1 Bell pepper, diced
- 3 Eggs, beaten
- 2 Tomatoes, chopped
- 1 tablespoon Hot sauce

Directions

- Grease the slow cooker with coconut oil from inside.
- Then mix hot sauce with beaten eggs.
- Add chopped tomatoes and bell pepper.
- Pour the mixture in the slow cooker and close the lid.
- Cook the meal on high for 2.5 hours.

Italian Style Scrambled Eggs

6 Servings

Preparation Time:4 hours 10 minutes

Ingredients

- ¼ cup Milk

- 1 teaspoon Italian seasonings

- ¼ teaspoon Salt

- 4 Eggs, beaten

- 3 oz Mozzarella, shredded

- 1 teaspoon Butter, melted

Directions

- Mix eggs with milk, Italian seasonings, and salt.

- Pour butter and milk mixture in the slow cooker and close the lid.

- Cook the meal on high for 1 hour.

- Then open the lid and scramble the eggs.

- After this, top the meal with cheese and cook the eggs on low for 3 hours more.

Egg Quiche

6 Servings

Preparation Time:7 hours 5 minutes

Ingredients

- 1 Onion, diced

- 1 teaspoon Chili flakes

- ½ teaspoon ground Paprika

- 4 Eggs, beaten

- 1 Bell pepper, diced

- 2 tablespoons Flax meal

Directions

- Mix eggs with flax meal.

- Add bell pepper, chili flakes, onion, and ground paprika.

- Pour the quiche mixture in the slow cooker and close the lid.

- Cook the meal on low for 7 hours.

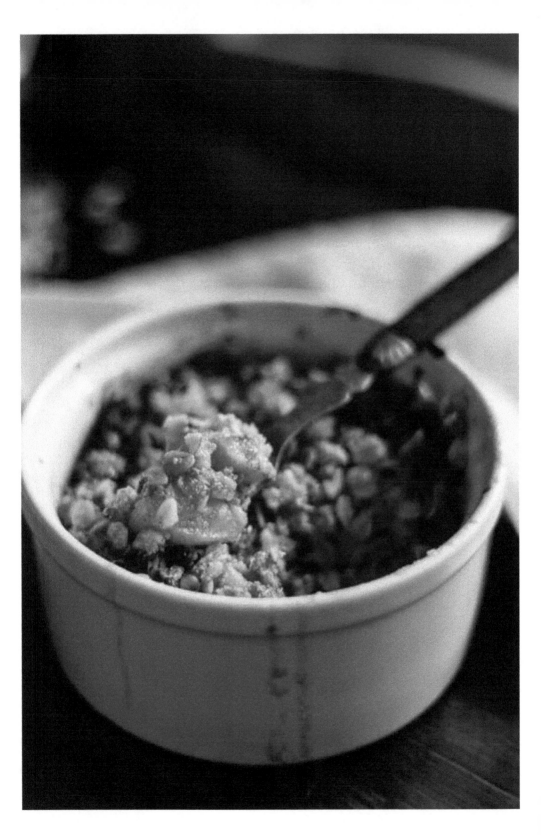

Basil Sausages

7 Servings

Preparation Time: 4 hours 10 minutes

Ingredients

- 1 teaspoon dried Basil

- 1 tablespoon Olive oil

- 1-pound Italian sausages, chopped

- 1 teaspoon ground Coriander

- ¼ cup of Water

Directions

- Sprinkle the chopped sausages with ground coriander and dried basil and transfer in the slow cooker.

- Add the olive oil and water.

- Close the lid and cook the sausages on high for 4 hours.

French toast

4 Servings

Preparation Time:3.5 hours 10 minutes

Ingredients

- 1 teaspoon white Sugar

- 1 Egg, beaten

- ¼ cup Milk

- 2 white Bread slices

- 1 teaspoon Cream cheese

- 1 tablespoon Butter

Directions

- Put butter in the slow cooker.

- Add cream cheese, white sugar, egg, and milk. Stir the mixture.

- Then put the bread slices in the slow cooker and close the lid.

- Cook the toasts for 3.5 hours on High.

Peach Oats

6 Servings

Preparation Time: 7 hours 10 minutes

Ingredients

- ½ cup Peaches, pitted, chopped

- ½ cup steel cut Oats

- 1 cup Milk

- 1 teaspoon ground Cardamom

Directions

- Mix steel-cut oats with milk and pour the mixture in the slow cooker.

- Add ground cardamom and peaches. Stir the ingredients gently and close the lid.

- Cook the meal on low for 7 hours.

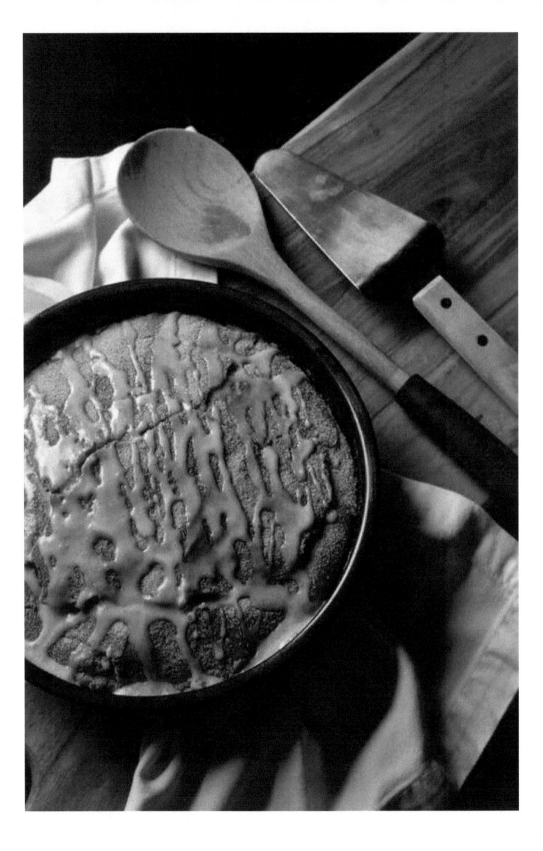

Shrimp Omelet

6 Servings

Preparation Time: 3.5 hours 8 minutes

Ingredients

- ½ teaspoon ground Turmeric
- ½ teaspoon ground Paprika
- ¼ teaspoon Salt
- 4 Eggs, beaten
- 4 oz Shrimps, peeled
- Cooking spray

Directions

- Mix eggs with shrimps, turmeric, salt, and paprika.
- Then spray the slow cooker bowl with cooking spray.
- After this, pour the egg mixture inside. Flatten the shrimps and close the lid.
- Cook the omelet for 3.5 hours on High.

Raisins and Rice Pudding

6 Servings

Preparation Time: 6 hours 5 minutes

Ingredients

- 2.5 cups organic Almond milk

- 2 tablespoons Cornstarch

- 1 teaspoon Vanilla extract

- 1 cup long-grain Rice

- 2 tablespoons Raisins, chopped

Directions

- Put all ingredients in the slow cooker and carefully mix.

- Then close the lid and cook the pudding for 6 hours on low.

LUNCH

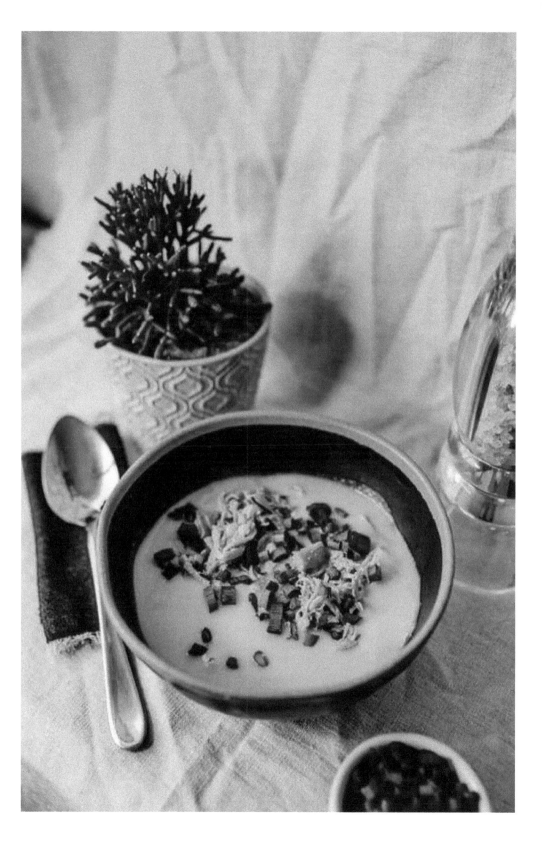

Barley-Stuffed Cabbage Rolls

6 Servings

Preparation Time: 3½ hours 15 minutes

Ingredients

- 3 ounces (85 g) feta Cheese, crumbled

- ½ cup dried Currants

- 2 tablespoons pine Nuts, toasted

- 2 tablespoons chopped fresh flat-leaf Parsley

- ½ teaspoon sea Salt, divided

- ½ teaspoon Black pepper, divided

- 1 large head green Cabbage, cored

- 1 tablespoon Olive oil

- 1 large yellow Onion, chopped

- 3 cups cooked pearl Barley

- ½ cup Apple juice

- 1 tablespoon Apple cider vinegar

- 1 (15-ounce / 425-g) can crushed Tomatoes, with the juice

Directions

- Steam the cabbage head in a large pot over boiling water for 8 minutes. Remove to a cutting board and let cool slightly.

- Remove 16 leaves from the cabbage head (reserve the rest of the cabbage for another use). Cut off the raised portion of the center vein of each cabbage leaf (do not cut out the vein).

- Heat the oil in a large nonstick lidded skillet over medium heat. Add the onion, cover, and cook 6 minutes or until tender. Remove to a large bowl.

- Stir the barley, feta cheese, currants, pine nuts, and parsley into the onion mixture. Season with ¼ teaspoon of the salt and ¼ teaspoon of the pepper.

- Place cabbage leaves on a work surface. On 1 cabbage leaf, spoon about ⅓ cup of the barley mixture into the center. Fold in the edges of the leaf over the barley mixture and roll the cabbage leaf up as if you were making a burrito. Repeat for the remaining 15 cabbage leaves and filling.

- Arrange the cabbage rolls in the slow cooker.

- Combine the remaining ¼ teaspoon salt, ¼ teaspoon pepper, the apple juice, apple cider vinegar, and tomatoes. Pour the apple juice mixture evenly over the cabbage rolls.

- Cover and cook on high for 2 hours or on low for 6 to 8 hours. Serve hot.

Sumptuous Chinese Vegetable Mix

8 Servings

Preparation Time: 3 to 6 hours 10 minutes

Ingredients

- 1 (8-ounce / 227-g) can water Chestnuts, drained

- 1 bunch Celery, sliced on the diagonal

- 1 large Onion, sliced

- 3 tablespoons Soy sauce

- 1 tablespoon Sugar

- 1 (12-ounce /340-g) package chop-suey vegetables

- 1 (1-pound / 454-g) can Bean sprouts, drained

- 2 (4-ounce / 113-g) cans sliced Mushrooms, drained

- ¼ teaspoon Black pepper, or to taste

- ¾ cup Water

- Cooking spray

Directions

- Spritz the slow cooker with cooking spray.

- Combine all ingredients in the slow cooker.

- Cover. Cook on low for 3 to 6 hours, depending upon how soft or crunchy you like the vegetables.

- Serve warm.

Papaya Salsa Swordfish

6 Servings

Preparation Time: 1 to 2 hour 15 minutes

Ingredients

- 2 tablespoons minced fresh cilantro, stems reserved

- ¼ cup dry white wine

- ¼ cup water

- 1 lime, sliced ¼ inch thick

- 4 (6- to 8-ounce / 170- to 227-g) skinless swordfish steaks, 1 to 1½ inches thick

- Salt and ground black pepper, to taste

Salsa

- 1 jalapeño chile, stemmed, deseeded, and minced

- 1 tablespoon extra-virgin olive oil

- ½ teaspoon lime zest

- 1 papaya, peeled, deseeded, and cut into ½-inch pieces

- 2 tablespoons lime juice

Directions

- Fold sheet of aluminum foil into sling and press widthwise into the slow cooker. Arrange lime slices in single layer in bottom of prepared slow cooker.

- Scatter cilantro stems over lime slices. Add wine to slow cooker, and then add water until liquid level is even with lime slices (about ¼ cup). Season swordfish with salt and pepper and arrange in even layer on top of cilantro stems.

- Cover and cook until swordfish flakes apart when gently prodded with a paring knife and registers 140ºF (60ºC), 1 to 2 hours on low.

- Mix papaya, jalapeño, oil, and lime zest and juice in a bowl. Season with salt and pepper to taste.

- Using sling, transfer swordfish to baking sheet. Gently lift and tilt steaks with a spatula to remove cilantro stems and lime slices. Transfer to serving dish.

- Discard poaching liquid and remove any white albumin from swordfish. Serve with salsa.

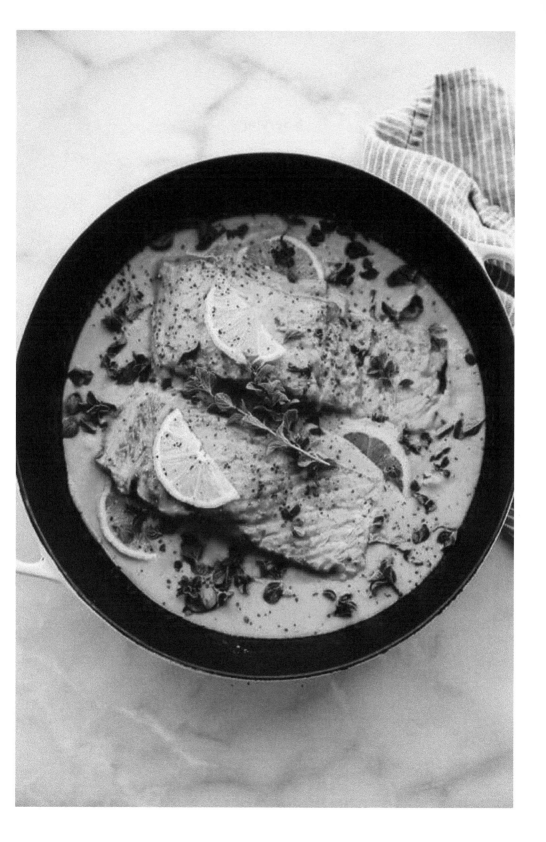

Hearty Cod Peperonata

6 Servings

Preparation Time: 1 to 2 hour 15 minutes

Ingredients

- 1 tablespoon paprika

- 2 teaspoons minced fresh thyme or ½ teaspoon dried

- ¼ teaspoon red pepper flakes

- Salt and ground black pepper, to taste

- 1 (14½-ounce / 411-g) can diced tomatoes, drained

- ¼ cup dry white wine

- 2 red or yellow bell peppers, stemmed, deseeded, and sliced thin

- 1 onion, halved and sliced thin

- 2 tablespoons extra-virgin olive oil, plus extra for drizzling

- 2 tablespoons tomato paste

- 4 garlic cloves, minced

- 4 (6- to 8-ounce / 170- to 227-g) skinless cod fillets, 1 to 1½ inches thick

- 2 tablespoons coarsely chopped fresh basil

- 2 teaspoons balsamic vinegar

Directions

- Microwave bell peppers, onion, oil, tomato paste, garlic, paprika, thyme, pepper flakes, ¼ teaspoon salt, and ¼ teaspoon pepper in a bowl, stirring occasionally, until vegetables are softened, about 8 minutes. Transfer to the slow cooker.

- Stir tomatoes and wine into the slow cooker. Season cod with salt and pepper and nestle into the slow cooker. Spoon portion of sauce over cod.

- Cover and cook until cod flakes apart when gently prodded with a paring knife and registers 140ºF (60ºC), 1 to 2 hours on low.

- Using 2 metal spatulas, transfer cod to serving dish. Stir basil and vinegar into sauce and season with salt and pepper to taste. Spoon sauce over cod and drizzle with extra oil. Serve warm.

Veracruz Flavor Slow Cooked Tilapia

8 Servings

Preparation Time: 2 to 4 hour 5 minutes

Ingredients

- 2 large tomatoes, chopped

- 1 large onion, chopped

- 1 bell pepper (any color), deseeded and thinly sliced

- ½ cup sliced pimento-stuffed green olives

- 4 garlic cloves, sliced

- 6 (6-ounce / 170-g) tilapia fillets

- 1 tablespoon olive oil

- ¼ teaspoon sea salt

- ½ teaspoon freshly ground black pepper

- 1 medium pepperoncino, deseeded and diced

- 2 tablespoons drained capers

- 6 lime wedges

- Cooking spray

Directions

- Spray the slow cooker with cooking spray.

- Brush the tilapia fillets with olive oil and sprinkle them lightly with salt and pepper. Lay the fillets on the bottom of the slow cooker.

- In a medium bowl, mix the tomatoes, onion, bell pepper, olives, garlic, pepperoncino, and capers. Then spoon this mixture over the fillets.

- Cover and cook on low for 2 to 4 hours, or until a meat thermometer inserted in the fish reads 145ºF (63ºC).

- Carefully remove the fillets to warm plates and spoon some vegetables and sauce over each before serving. Garnish with lime wedges.

Asian Napa Cabbage Wraps

6 Servings

Preparation Time: 1½ to 2 hours 15 minutes

Ingredients

- 4 slices fresh ginger
- 2 tablespoons vegetable oil
- 2 cloves garlic, minced
- 1 teaspoon freshly grated ginger
- 6 canned water chestnuts, finely chopped
- 2 chicken breast halves, skin and bones removed, finely chopped
- 4 green onions, finely chopped, using the white and tender green parts
- 2 tablespoons hoisin sauce
- 1 head Napa cabbage
- 2 cups chicken broth
- ½ cup soy sauce
- 1 tablespoon cornstarch mixed with 2 tablespoons water

Directions

- Core the cabbage and separate the leaves, being careful not to tear them. Put the broth, soy sauce, and ginger in a large stockpot and bring to a boil.

- Blanch the cabbage leaves, one at a time, for 30 seconds until limp. Drain the leaves and set aside. Add the broth mixture to a slow cooker. Cover and set on warm while preparing the filling.

- Heat the oil in a sauté pan over high heat. Add the garlic, ginger, and water chestnuts and sauté for 30 seconds. Add the chicken and cook until the chicken turns white, for 3 to 5 minutes.

- Transfer the contents of the pan to a bowl and stir in the green onions and hoisin sauce. Place 2 to 3 tablespoons of filling at the stem end of a cabbage leaf and roll up, tucking in the sides of the leaf as you go. Place the cabbage wraps on a rack in the slow cooker.

- Cover and cook on high for 1½ to 2 hours, until the chicken is cooked through. Remove the wraps and set aside. Strain the broth through a fine-mesh sieve into a saucepan and bring to a boil. Add the cornstarch mixture and bring back to a boil.

- Serve the wraps with the sauce on the side.

Chicken with Broccoli and Miso

8 Servings

Preparation Time: 1½ to 2 hours 10 minutes

Ingredients

- 1 clove garlic, sliced
- 2 thin slices fresh ginger
- 6 chicken breast halves, skin and bones removed
- 2 cups chicken broth
- ¼ cup white miso paste
- 1 pound (454 g) broccoli, stalks trimmed and peeled and cut into florets

Directions

- Pour the broth into a slow cooker. Add the miso, garlic, and ginger and stir to combine.
- Place the chicken in the broth and place the broccoli on top of the chicken. Cover and cook on high for 1½ to 2 hours, until the chicken is cooked through and the broccoli is tender.
- Remove the chicken from the broth and arrange it on a serving platter, surrounded by the broccoli. Strain the broth through a fine-mesh sieve and serve in bowls. The chicken can also be served in bowls.

Balsamic Chicken with Figs

8 Servings

Preparation Time: 2¼ hours 10 minutes

Ingredients

- ½ teaspoon freshly ground black pepper
- ½ cup balsamic vinegar
- ½ cup Ruby Port
- ½ cup chicken broth
- 1 teaspoon dried thyme
- 16 dried figs, cut in half
- 2 tablespoons vegetable oil
- 8 chicken breast halves, skin and bones removed
- 1½ teaspoons salt

Directions

- Heat the oil in a large skillet over medium-high heat. Sprinkle the chicken evenly with the salt and pepper.

- Add the chicken to the skillet and brown on all sides, for 12 to 15 minutes.

- Transfer the chicken to a slow cooker. Deglaze the skillet with the vinegar and port, scraping up any browned bits from the bottom of the skillet. Add the broth and transfer the contents of the skillet to the slow cooker.

- Add the thyme and figs and stir to combine. Cover and cook on high for 2 hours, until the chicken is cooked through and the sauce is syrupy.

- Serve warm.

SNACKS AND SIDES

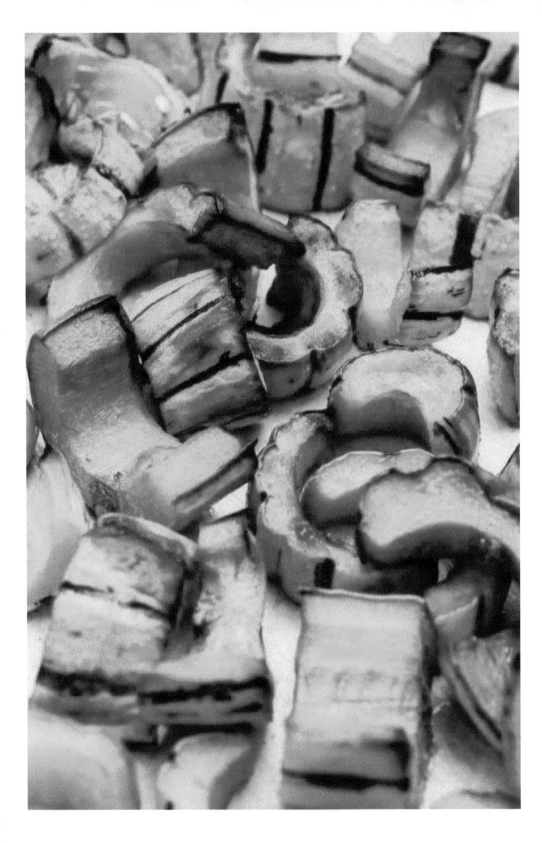

Herbed Mashed Potatoes

8 Servings

Preparation Time: 2 to 3 hours 15 minutes

Ingredients

- 3 tablespoons minced Chives
- 3 Garlic cloves, minced
- 1 tablespoon minced fresh Parsley
- 1 teaspoon minced fresh Thyme
- ½ teaspoon Salt
- ¼ teaspoon Pepper
- 4 pounds (1.8 kg) Yukon Gold potatoes (about 12 medium), peeled and cubed
- 1 (8-ounce / 227-g) package Cream cheese, softened and cubed
- 1 cup Sour cream
- ½ cup Butter, cubed
- ⅓ cup Heavy whipping cream

Directions

- Place the potatoes in a Dutch oven and cover with water. Bring to a boil.

- Reduce heat. Cover and cook for 10 to 15 minutes or until tender. Drain.

- Mash the potatoes with the cream cheese, sour cream, butter and cream. Stir in the remaining ingredients.

- Transfer to a greased slow cooker. Cover and cook on low for 2 to 3 hours or until heated through.

- Serve warm.

Creamy Potato Mash

8 Servings

Preparation Time: 3 to 3 ½ hours 15 minutes

Ingredients

- ½ teaspoon Garlic powder
- 3 pounds (1.4 kg) potatoes (about 9 medium), peeled and cubed
- 1 (8-ounce / 227-g) package cream cheese, softened
- 1 cup sour cream
- ½ cup butter, cubed
- ¼ cup 2% milk
- 1½ cups shredded Cheddar cheese
- 1½ cups shredded Pepper Jack cheese
- ½ pound (227 g) bacon strips, cooked and crumbled
- 4 green onions, chopped
- ½ teaspoon onion powder

Directions

- Place the potatoes in a Dutch oven and cover with water. Bring to a boil.

- Reduce heat. Cover and cook for 10 to 15 minutes or until tender. Drain.

- Mash the potatoes with the cream cheese, sour cream, butter and milk.

- Stir in the cheeses, bacon, onions and seasonings. Transfer to a large bowl. Cover and refrigerate overnight.

- Transfer to a greased slow cooker. Cover and cook on low for 3 to 3 ½ hours.

- Serve hot.

Hash Brown Potatoes in Cream

8 Servings

Preparation Time: 3 ½ to 4 hours 5 minutes

Ingredients

- 1 cup sour cream
- ¼ teaspoon pepper
- ⅛ teaspoon salt
- 1 (8-ounce / 227-g) carton spreadable chive and onion cream cheese
- 1 (32-ounce / 907-g) package frozen cubed hash brown potatoes, thawed
- 1 (10¾-ounce / 305-g) can condensed cream of potato soup, undiluted
- 2 cups shredded Colby-Monterey Jack cheese

Directions

- Place the potatoes in a lightly greased slow cooker.
- In a large bowl, combine the soup, cheese, sour cream, pepper and salt. Pour over the potatoes and mix well.
- Cover and cook on low for 3 ½ to 4 hours or until potatoes are tender. Stir in the cream cheese.

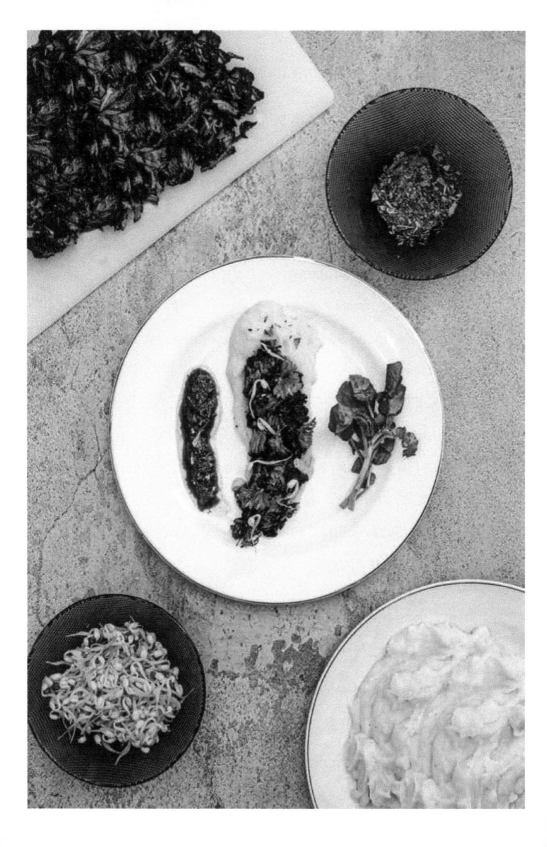

Hash Brown Potato Casserole

6 Servings

Preparation Time: 3 ¼ to 4 ½ hours 5 minutes

Ingredients

- 1 (32-ounce / 907-g) package frozen cubed hash brown potatoes, thawed
- 1 (10¾-ounce / 305-g) can condensed cream of celery soup, undiluted
- 1 (10¾-ounce / 305-g) can condensed nacho cheese soup, undiluted
- 1 large onion, finely chopped
- ⅓ cup butter, melted
- 1 cup reduced-fat sour cream

Directions

- In a greased slow cooker, combine the first five ingredients.
- Cover and cook on low for 3 to 4 hours or until potatoes are tender.
- Stir in the sour cream. Cover and cook for 15 to 30 minutes longer or until heated through. Serve warm.

Potato and Black Bean Gratin

8 Servings

Preparation Time: 8 to 10 hours 15 minutes

Ingredients

- 2 garlic cloves, minced
- 1 teaspoon dried thyme
- ¼ teaspoon coarsely ground pepper
- 1½ pounds (680 g) medium red potatoes, cut into ¼-inch slices
- 1 teaspoon salt
- 1 cup shredded Cheddar cheese
- 2 (15-ounce / 425-g) cans black beans, rinsed and drained
- 1 (10¾-ounce / 305-g) can condensed cream of mushroom soup, undiluted
- 1 medium sweet red pepper, chopped
- 1 cup frozen peas, thawed
- 1 cup chopped sweet onion
- 1 celery rib, thinly sliced

Directions

- In a large bowl, combine the beans, soup, red pepper, peas, onion, celery, garlic, thyme and pepper.

- Spoon half of the mixture into a greased slow cooker. Layer with half of the potatoes, salt and cheese. Repeat layers.

- Cover and cook on low for 8 to 10 hours or until potatoes are tender.

- Serve hot.

Spicy BBQ Beans and Corn

8 Servings

Preparation Time: 5to 6 hours 10 minutes

Ingredients

- 1 (16-ounce / 454-g) can kidney beans, rinsed and drained
- 1 (15¼-ounce / 432-g) can whole kernel corn, drained
- 1 (15-ounce / 425-g) can garbanzo beans or chickpeas, rinsed and drained
- 1 (15-ounce / 425-g) can black beans, rinsed and drained
- 1 (15-ounce / 425-g) can chili with beans
- 1 cup barbecue sauce
- 1 cup salsa
- ⅓ cup packed brown sugar
- ¼ teaspoon hot pepper sauce
- Chopped green onions (optional)

Directions

- In a slow cooker, combine the first nine ingredients. Cover and cook on low for 5 to 6 hours.
- Serve topped with the green onions, if desired.

Braised Beans and Bacon

8 Servings

Preparation Time: 6 to 8 hours 15 minutes

Ingredients

- 1 (15¼-ounce / 432-g) can lima beans, rinsed and drained
- 1 (15-ounce / 425-g) can black beans, rinsed and drained
- 1 cup packed brown sugar
- ½ cup cider vinegar
- 1 tablespoon molasses
- 2 teaspoons garlic powder
- ½ teaspoon ground mustard
- 1 (1-pound / 454-g) package sliced bacon, chopped
- 1 cup chopped onion
- 2 (15-ounce / 425-g) cans pork and beans, undrained
- 1 (16-ounce / 454-g) can kidney beans, rinsed and drained
- 1 (16-ounce / 454-g) can butter beans, rinsed and drained

Directions

- In a large skillet, cook the bacon and onion over medium heat for 4 minutes, until the bacon is crisp. Remove to paper towels to drain.

- In a slow cooker, combine the remaining ingredients. Stir in the bacon mixture. Cover and cook on low for 6 to 8 hours or until heated through.

- Serve hot.

Tangy Banana-Raisin Applesauce

7 cups Servings

Preparation Time: 3 to 4 hours 10 minutes

Ingredients

- ¼ cup butter, melted
- 2 teaspoons pumpkin pie spice
- 1 small lemon
- 1 envelope instant apples and cinnamon oatmeal
- ½ cup boiling water
- 8 medium apples, peeled and cubed
- 1 medium ripe banana, thinly sliced
- 1 cup raisins
- ¾ cup orange juice
- ½ cup packed brown sugar
- ¼ cup honey
- Cooking spray

Directions

- Place the apples, banana and raisins in a slow cooker coated with cooking spray.

- In a small bowl, combine the orange juice, brown sugar, honey, butter and pie spice. Pour over apple mixture.

- Cut ends off lemon. Cut into six wedges and remove the seeds. Transfer to the slow cooker.

- Cover and cook on high for 3 to 4 hours or until apples are soft.

- Discard the lemon. Mash the apple mixture. In a small bowl, combine the oatmeal and water. Let stand for 1 minute. Stir into the applesauce. Serve.

Sweet Green Beans with Bacon

8 Servings

Preparation Time: 4 ½ hours 10 minutes

Ingredients

- 1 (28-ounce / 794-g) can petite diced tomatoes, undrained
- ¼ cup packed brown sugar
- 1 tablespoon seasoned pepper
- ½ teaspoon seasoned salt
- 1 (16-ounce / 454-g) can red beans, rinsed and drained
- 1 (14-ounce / 397-g) package thick-sliced bacon strips, chopped
- 1 large red onion, chopped
- 2 (16-ounce / 454-g) packages frozen cut green beans, thawed

Directions

- In a large skillet, cook the bacon over medium heat for 3 minutes, until partially cooked but not crisp, stirring occasionally.

- Remove with a slotted spoon and drain on paper towels. Discard the drippings, reserving 2 tablespoons.

- Add the onion to the drippings. Cook and stir over medium-high heat for 4 minutes or until tender.

- In a slow cooker, combine the green beans, tomatoes, brown sugar, pepper, salt, bacon and onion. Cook, covered, on low for 4 hours. Stir in the red beans.

- Cook for 30 minutes longer or until heated through.

- Serve warm.

DINNER

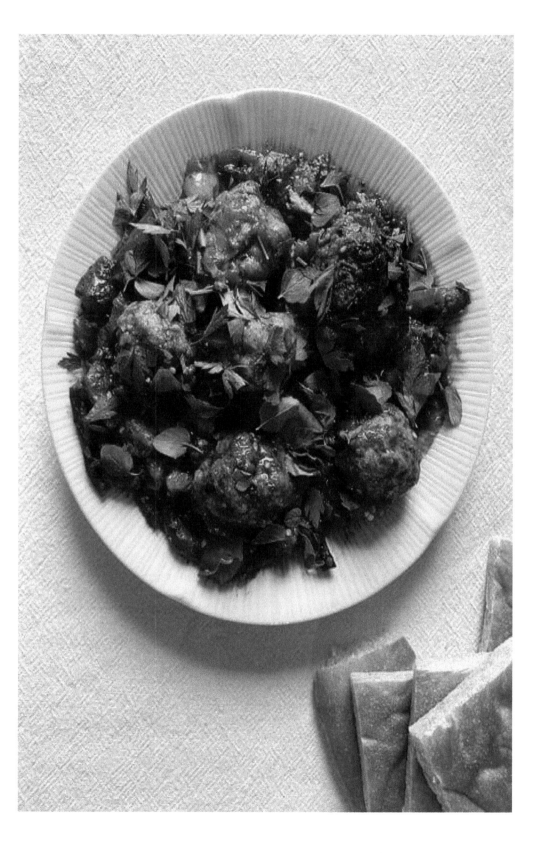

Braised California Chicken

8 Servings

Preparation Time: 8½ to 9½ hours 10 minutes

Ingredients

- 1 teaspoon dry mustard
- 1 teaspoon garlic salt
- 2 tablespoons chopped green peppers
- 3 medium oranges, peeled and separated into slices
- 3 pounds (1.4 kg) chicken, quartered
- 1 cup orange juice
- ⅓ cup chili sauce
- 2 tablespoons soy sauce
- 1 tablespoon molasses

Directions

- Arrange the chicken in a slow cooker.
- In a bowl, combine the orange juice, chili sauce, soy sauce, molasses, dry mustard, and garlic salt. Pour over the chicken.
- Cover. Cook on low for 8 to 9 hours.
- Stir in the green peppers and oranges. Cook for 30 minutes longer. Serve warm.

Beef Braised in Barolo

8 Servings

Preparation Time: 4 hours 10 minutes

Ingredients

- 4 pounds (1.8 kg) beef chuck, cut into 1-inch pieces
- 2 large sweet onions, cut into half rounds
- 2 teaspoons sugar
- 1 tablespoon crushed dried rosemary
- ½ cup red wine, such as Chianti or Barolo
- 4 tablespoons olive oil, divided
- Salt and freshly ground black pepper, to taste
- 3 cloves garlic, minced
- 1 (32-ounce / 907-g) can crushed tomatoes, with the juice

Directions

- Put 2 tablespoons of the oil, 1½ teaspoons salt, ½ teaspoon pepper, and the garlic in a small bowl and stir to combine. Add the meat to the bowl and toss to coat in the mixture.

- Heat the remaining 2 tablespoons of the oil in a large skillet over high heat.

- Add the beef and brown on all sides for 4 minutes. Transfer to a slow cooker insert. Add the onions, sugar, and rosemary to the same skillet over medium-high heat and sauté until the onions begin to soften, for 3 to 4 minutes.

- Transfer the contents of the skillet to the slow cooker insert. Add the wine and tomatoes and stir to combine. Cover and cook on high for 4 hours or on low for 8 hours until the beef is tender. Remove the beef from the slow cooker with a slotted spoon and cover with aluminum foil.

- Skim off the fat from the top of the sauce and season with salt and pepper.

- Serve the beef with the sauce on a platter.

North African Beef and Bean Stew

6 Servings

Preparation Time: 8⅓ to 10½ hours 15 minutes

Ingredients

- 2 cloves garlic, sliced
- 4 medium carrots, coarsely chopped
- 2 teaspoons sweet paprika
- 1 teaspoon ground cumin
- ½ teaspoon ground cinnamon
- 3 cups beef broth, divided
- 1 (15-ounce / 425-g) can garbanzo beans, drained and rinsed
- 1 cup dried apricots, cut into ½-inch pieces
- ½ cup golden raisins
- 3 tablespoons olive oil
- 3 pounds (1.4 kg) beef chuck roast, cut into 1-inch pieces
- 1½ teaspoons salt
- 1 teaspoon freshly ground black pepper
- 1 large onion, coarsely chopped
- 2 tablespoons cornstarch mixed with ¼ cup water

Directions

- Heat the oil in a large skillet over high heat. Sprinkle the meat evenly with the salt and pepper. Add the meat to the skillet a few pieces at a time and brown on all sides for 4 minutes. Transfer the browned meat to the insert of a slow cooker.

- Add the onion and garlic to the same skillet and sauté until the onion begins to soften, for about 3 minutes. Add the carrots, paprika, cumin, and cinnamon and sauté until the spices are fragrant, for about 2 minutes.

- Deglaze the skillet with 1 cup of the broth and scrape up any browned bits from the bottom of the pan. Transfer the contents of the skillet to the slow cooker insert. Add the remaining 2 cups of the broth, the beans, apricots, and raisins.

- Cover the slow cooker and cook on low for 8 to 10 hours, until the meat is tender.

- Skim off any fat from the top of the stew. Add the cornstarch mixture and stir to combine. Cover the slow cooker and cook for an additional 20 to 30 minutes until the sauce is thickened.

- Serve the stew warm from the cooker.

Slow Cooked Tex-Mex Chicken and Rice

6 Servings

Preparation Time: 4 to 4½ hours 15 minutes

Ingredients

- 4 whole boneless, skinless chicken breasts, cut into ½-inch cubes
- 2 medium onions, chopped
- 1 green pepper, chopped
- 1 (4-ounce / 113-g) can diced green chilies
- 1 teaspoon garlic powder
- ½ teaspoon pepper
- 1 cup uncooked converted white rice
- 1 (28-ounce / 794-g) can diced peeled tomatoes
- 1 (6-ounce / 170-g) can tomato paste
- 3 cups hot water
- 1 package dry taco seasoning mix

Directions

- Combine all the ingredients, except for the chilies and seasonings, in a slow cooker.

- Cover. Cook on low for 4 to 4½ hours, or until the rice is tender and the chicken is cooked.

- Stir in the green chilies and seasonings and serve.

Mushroom and Tomato Mussels

6 Servings

Preparation Time: 2½ to 3½ hours 15 minutes

Ingredients

- 8 ounces (227 g) mushrooms, diced
- 1 (28-ounce / 794-g) can diced tomatoes, with the juice
- ¾ cup white wine
- 2 tablespoons dried oregano
- ½ tablespoon dried basil
- 3 tablespoons olive oil
- 4 cloves garlic, minced
- 3 shallot cloves, minced
- ½ teaspoon black pepper
- 1 teaspoon paprika
- ¼ teaspoon red pepper flakes
- 3 pounds (1.4 kg) mussels

Directions

- In a large sauté pan, heat the olive oil over medium-high heat. Cook the garlic, shallots, and mushrooms for 2 to 3 minutes, until the garlic is brown and fragrant. Scrape the entire contents of the pan into the slow cooker.

- Add the tomatoes and white wine to the slow cooker. Sprinkle with the oregano, basil, black pepper, paprika, and red pepper flakes.
- Cover and cook on low for 4 to 5 hours or on high for 2 to 3 hours. The mixture is done cooking when mushrooms are fork-tender.
- Clean and debeard the mussels. Discard any open mussels.
- Increase the heat on the slow cooker to high once the mushroom mixture is done. Add the cleaned mussels to the slow cooker and secure the lid tightly. Cook for 30 more minutes.
- To serve, ladle the mussels into bowls with plenty of broth. Discard any mussels that didn't open up during cooking. Serve hot, with crusty bread for sopping up the sauce.

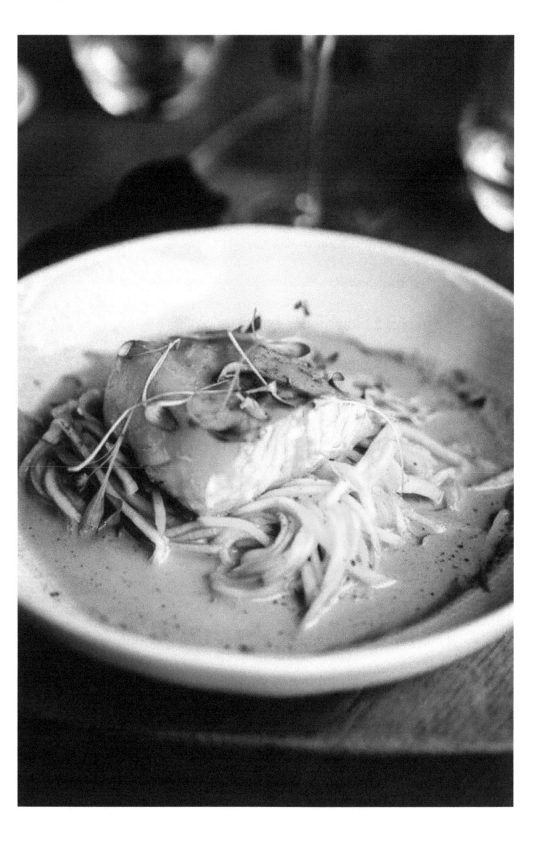

Spanish Herbed Octopus

4 Servings

Preparation Time: 1¼ hours hour 15 minutes

Ingredients

- 1 bunch fresh oregano

- 2 dried bay leaves

- ¼ cup plus 2 tablespoons extra-virgin olive oil

- Coarse salt, to taste

- 2 garlic cloves, minced

- 2 pounds (907 g) octopus, cleaned

- 1 small fennel, trimmed, bulb and fronds coarsely chopped

- 2 small onions, thickly sliced

- 1 bunch fresh flat-leaf parsley

- ¼ cup capers, drained, rinsed, and coarsely chopped

- Juice of 2 lemons (about ⅓ cup)

- ¼ teaspoon hot smoked paprika

- ¼ teaspoon sweet smoked paprika

Directions

- Bring a large stockpot of water to a boil. Add octopus and boil briefly to tenderize, about 2 minutes. Drain and let cool, then slice octopus into 2-inch pieces.

- Place fennel, onions, parsley, oregano, and bay leaves in the slow cooker. Arrange octopus over vegetables. Drizzle with 1 tablespoon oil and ½ teaspoon salt. Cover and cook on low until octopus is tender, 2 hours, or on high for 1 hour.

- Heat a grill or grill pan to High. Remove octopus and half the vegetables from the slow cooker (discard remaining vegetables and liquid). Toss with 1 tablespoon oil and grill until charred, about 6 minutes. Transfer to a bowl.

- Meanwhile, gently heat remaining ¼ cup oil in a small skillet. Add garlic and cook until just fragrant, about 2 minutes. Stir in capers and lemon juice.

- Remove from heat and stir in both paprikas. Pour over octopus, toss, season with salt, and serve.

Garlicky Northern Beans

8 Servings

Preparation Time: 6 to 8 hours 15 minutes

Ingredients

- 1 large sprig fresh rosemary
- ½ teaspoon salt
- ⅛ teaspoon white pepper
- 4 cups water
- 1 pound (454 g) great northern beans, rinsed and drained
- 1 onion, finely chopped
- 3 cloves garlic, minced
- 2 cups vegetable broth

Directions

- Combine the beans, onion, garlic, rosemary, salt, water, and vegetable broth in the slow cooker.
- Cover and cook on low for 6 to 8 hours or until the beans are tender.
- Remove the rosemary stem and discard. Stir the mixture gently and serve.

French White Beans

4 Servings

Preparation Time: 6 to 7 hours 10 minutes

Ingredients

- 3 garlic cloves, minced

- 3 cups chicken stock or vegetable broth

- ½ teaspoon dried thyme leaves

- 1 teaspoon salt

- ⅛ teaspoon freshly ground black pepper

- 2 tablespoons extra-virgin olive oil

- 1½ cups dried great northern beans, sorted and rinsed

- 2 carrots, sliced

- 1 onion, chopped

- 1 tablespoon minced fresh thyme leaves

- ⅓ cup grated Parmesan cheese

Directions

- In the slow cooker, combine all the ingredients except the fresh thyme and cheese, and stir.

- Cover and cook on low for 6 to 7 hours, or until the beans are tender.

- Stir in the fresh thyme and cheese, and serve.

Savory and Sweet Brisket

8 Servings

Preparation Time: 8 to 10 hours 10 minutes

Ingredients

- 1 cup ketchup
- ¼ cup grape jelly
- 1 envelope dry onion soup mix
- 3 to 3½ pounds (1.4 to 1.5 kg) fresh beef brisket, cut in half, divided
- ½ teaspoon pepper

Directions

- Place half of the brisket in a slow cooker.
- In a bowl, combine the ketchup, jelly, dry soup mix, and pepper.
- Spread half the mixture over half the meat. Top with the remaining meat and then the remaining ketchup mixture.
- Cover and cook on low for 8 to 10 hours or until meat is tender but not dry.
- Allow meat to rest for 10 minutes. Then slice and serve with the cooking juices

STEW & CHILIES

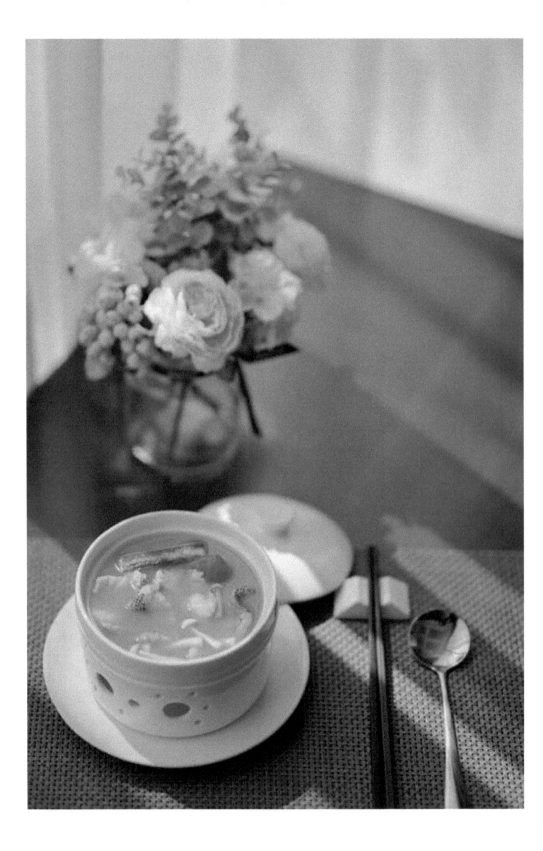

Meat Baby Carrot Stew

5 Servings

Preparation Time: 8 hours 10 minutes

Ingredients

- 1 teaspoon Peppercorns

- 3 cups of Water

- 1 bay Leaf

- 1 cup Baby carrot

- 6 oz Lamb loin, chopped

- 1 tablespoon Tomato paste

Directions

- Put all ingredients in the slow cooker.

- Close the lid and cook the stew on low for 8 hours.

- Carefully stir the stew and cool it to the room temperature.

Pumpkin Stew with Chicken

4 Servings

Preparation Time: 4 hours 10 minutes

Ingredients

- ¼ cup Coconut cream
- ½ teaspoon ground Cinnamon
- 1 Onion, chopped
- ½ cup Pumpkin, chopped
- 6 oz Chicken fillet, cut into strips
- 1 tablespoon Curry powder

Directions

- Mix pumpkin with chicken fillet strips in the mixing bowl.
- Add curry powder, coconut cream, ground cinnamon, and onion.
- Mix the stew ingredients and transfer them in the slow cooker.
- Cook the meal on high for 4 hours.

Ginger Fish Stew

7 Servings

Preparation Time: 6 hours 10 minutes

Ingredients

- 1 teaspoon Fish sauce

- ½ teaspoon ground Nutmeg

- ½ cup Green peas

- 3 cups of Water

- 1 oz fresh Ginger, peeled, chopped

- 1 cup Baby carrot

- 1-pound Salmon fillet, chopped

Directions

- Put all ingredients in the slow cooker bowl.

- Gently stir the stew ingredients and close the lid.

- Cook the stew on low for 6 hours.

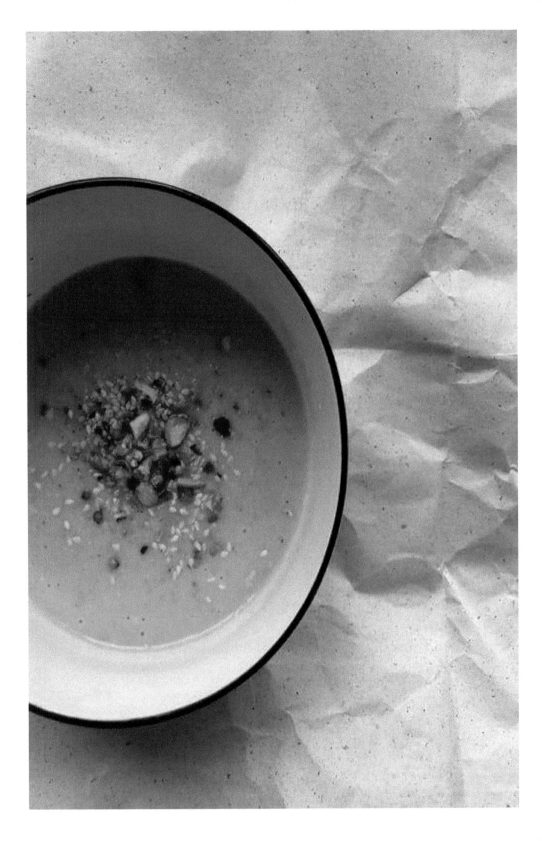

Mexican Style Stew

8 Servings

Preparation Time: 6 hours 10 minutes

Ingredients

- 4 cups Chicken stock

- 1 teaspoon Taco seasoning

- 1 teaspoon dried Cilantro

- 1 tablespoon Butter

- 1 cup Corn kernels

- 1 cup Green peas

- ¼ cup white Rice

Directions

- Put butter and wild rice in the slow cooker.

- Then add corn kernels, green peas, chicken stock, taco seasoning, and dried cilantro.

- Close the lid and cook the stew on low for 6 hours.

Mussel Stew

6 Servings

Preparation Time: 60 minutes

Ingredients

- 1 Eggplant, chopped

- 1 cup Coconut cream

- 1 tablespoon Sesame seeds

- 1 teaspoon Tomato paste

- 1-pound Mussels

- 2 Garlic cloves, diced

- 1 teaspoon Smoked paprika

- ½ teaspoon Chili powder

Directions

- Put all ingredients from the list above in the slow cooker and gently stir.

- Cover the lid and cook the mussel stew for 55 minutes on High.

Chinese Style Cod Stew

4 Servings

Preparation Time: 5 hours10 minutes

Ingredients

- 1 Garlic clove, chopped

- ¼ cup of Soy sauce

- ¼ cup Fish stock

- 4 oz Fennel bulb, chopped

- 6 oz Cod fillet

- 1 teaspoon Sesame seeds

- 1 teaspoon Olive oil

Directions

- Pour fish stock in the slow cooker.

- Add soy sauce, olive oil, garlic, and sesame seeds.

- Then chop the fish roughly and add in the slow cooker.

- Cook the meal on low for 5 hours.

Taco Spices Stew

6 Servings

Preparation Time: 8 hours10 minutes

Ingredients

- 1 cup Sweet potato, chopped

- 1 teaspoon Salt

- 1 teaspoon Taco seasonings

- 1-pound Beef sirloin

- 1 teaspoon liquid Honey

- 3 cups of Water

Directions

- Cut the beef sirloin into the strips and sprinkle with taco seasonings.

- Then transfer the beef strips in the slow cooker.

- Add salt, sweet potato, water, and liquid honey.

- Close the lid and cook the stew for 8 hours on low.

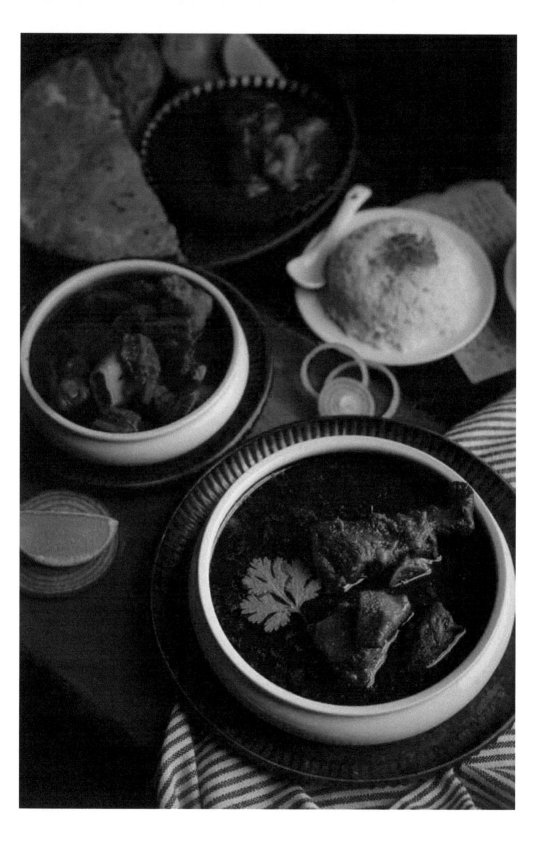

Crab Stew

6 Servings

Preparation Time: 5 hours10 minutes

Ingredients

- 1 teaspoon ground Turmeric

- 1 Potato, peeled chopped

- 1 cup of Water

- ½ cup of Coconut milk

- 8 oz Crab meat, chopped

- ½ cup Mango, chopped

- 1 teaspoon dried Lemongrass

Directions

- Put all ingredients in the slow cooker.

- Gently stir them with the help of the spoon and close the lid.

- Cook the stew on low for 5 hours.

- Then leave the cooked stew for 10-15 minutes to rest.

DESSERTS

Caramel Pie

6 Servings

Preparation Time: 2 hours 15 minutes

Ingredients

- 1 teaspoon butter, melted
- 4 caramels, candy, crushed
- 1 cup vanilla cake mix
- 4 eggs, beaten

Direction

- Mix vanilla cake mix with eggs and butter.
- Pour the liquid in the slow cooker and sprinkle with crushed candies.
- Close the lid and cook the pie on high for 2 hours.
- Then cool it and remove from the slow cooker.
- Cut the pie into 6 servings.

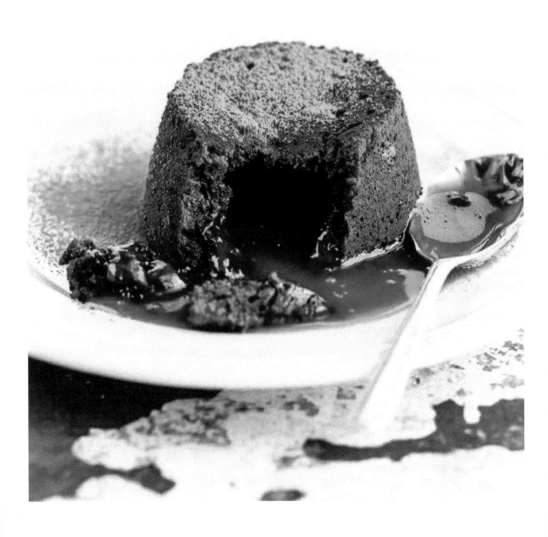

Blueberry Tapioca Pudding

4 Servings

Preparation Time: 3 hours 10 minutes

Ingredients

- 2 cups of milk

- 4 teaspoons blueberry jam

- 4 tablespoons tapioca

Direction

- Mix tapioca with milk and pour it in the slow cooker.

- Close the lid and cook the liquid on low for 3 hours.

- Then put the blueberry jam in 4 ramekins.

- Cool the cooked tapioca pudding until warm and pour over the jam.

Soft Thin Pie

6 Servings

Preparation Time: 2 hours 15 minutes

Ingredients

- 1 teaspoon vanilla extract
- ¼ cup of coconut oil
- ½ teaspoon baking powder
- 1 cup coconut flour
- ½ cup coconut flakes
- 3 eggs, beaten
- ¼ cup of sugar

Direction

- In the bowl, mix coconut flour, coconut flakes, eggs, sugar, vanilla extract, and baking powder.
- Add coconut oil and stir the mixture until homogenous.
- Then line the slow cooker bowl with baking paper and put the dough inside.
- Flatten it and close the lid.
- Cook the pie on High for 2 hours.
- Then cool it well and cut into serving bars.

Orange Cake

12 Servings

Preparation Time: 2 hours 20 minutes

Ingredients

- 2 cups semolina

- ½ cup of sugar

- 2 cups of orange juice

- ½ cup poppy seeds

- ½ cup olive oil

Direction

- Mix orange juice with poppy seeds, olive oil, sugar, and semolina.

- Then pour the liquid in the slow cooker.

- Cook it on High for 2 hours.

- When the cooking time is finished, let the cake to cool to the room temperature, remove it from the slow cooker and cut into servings.

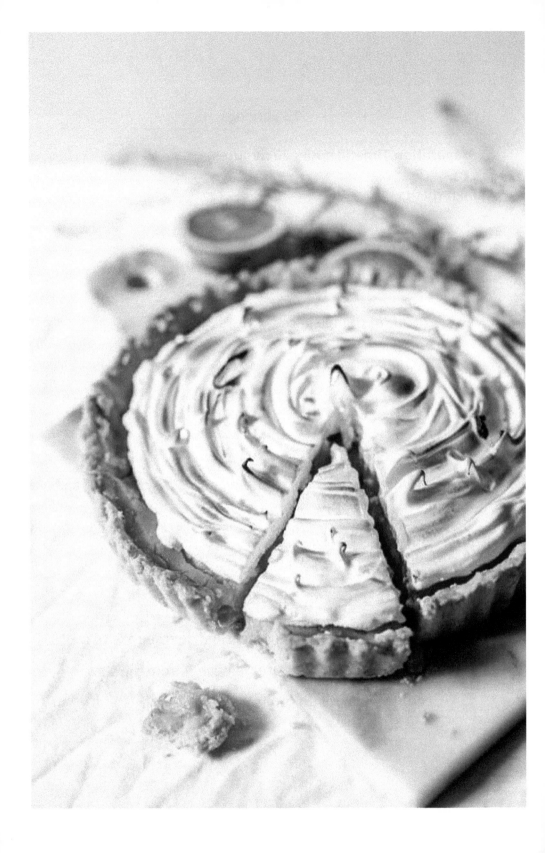

Pavlova

6 Servings

Preparation Time: 3 hours 15 minutes

Ingredients

- 1 teaspoon lemon juice

- 1 teaspoon vanilla extract

- 5 eggs' white

- 1 cup of sugar powder

- ½ cup whipped cream

Direction

- Mix egg whites with sugar powder, lemon juice, and vanilla extract and whisk until you get firm peaks.

- Then line the slow cooker with baking paper and put the egg white mixture inside.

- Flatten it and cook for 3 hours on low.

- When the egg white mixture is cooked, transfer it in the serving plate and top with whipped cream.

Peach Bread Pudding

6 Servings

Preparation Time: 6 hours 10 minutes

Ingredients

- 5 oz white bread, chopped

- 2 eggs, beaten

- 1 cup heavy cream

- ½ cup peaches, chopped

- 1 teaspoon flour

- 1 teaspoon coconut oil

- 2 tablespoons sugar

Directions

- Grease the slow cooker bottom with coconut oil.

- Then add white bread.

- Mix heavy cream with eggs, flour, sugar, and pour over the bread.

- Then add peaches and close the lid.

- Cook the pudding on low for 6 hours.

Almond Bars

6 Servings

Preparation Time: 2 hours 15 minutes

Ingredients

- 2 oz almonds, chopped

- ¼ cup of sugar

- 2 eggs, beaten

- 1 tablespoon cocoa powder

- ½ cup flour

- ½ cup coconut flour

- 4 tablespoons coconut oil

- 1 teaspoon baking powder

Direction

- Mix all ingredients in the bowl and knead the smooth dough.

- Then put the dough in the slow cooker, flatten it, and cut into bars.

- Close the lid and cook the dessert on High for 2 hours.

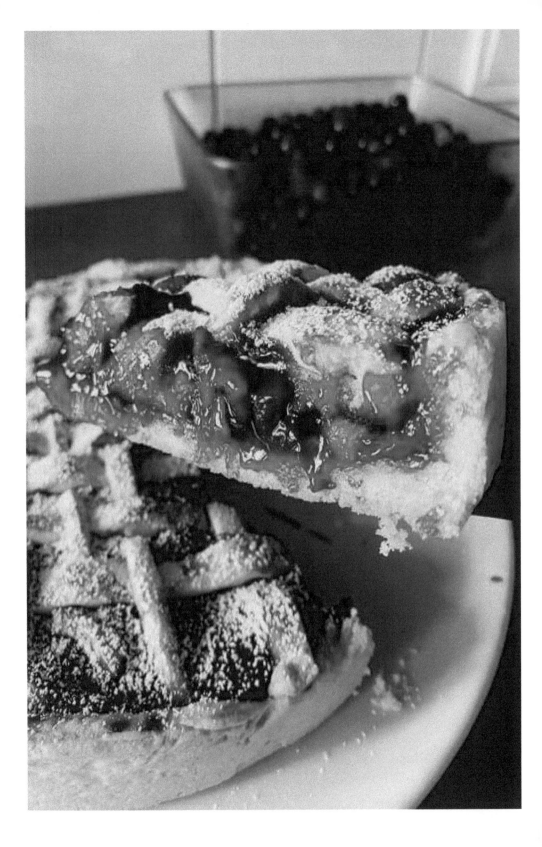

Caramel

10 Servings

Preparation Time: 7 hours 10 minutes

Ingredients

- 1 cup heavy cream

- 2 tablespoons butter

- 1 cup of sugar

Direction

- Put sugar in the slow cooker.

- Add heavy cream and butter.

- Close the lid and cook the caramel on low for 7 hours.

- Carefully mix the cooked caramel and transfer it in the glass cans.